An Extensive Body Reshape:

"Your Weight-Loss Plan for a Flat Belly and Optimal Health"

by

Mark T.Riggs

Table of contents

Description

Stop — and, surprisingly, turn around! — age-related weight gain and muscle misfortune with the very first weight reduction plan explicitly intended to shrivel your tummy, expand your life, and make your best self at midlife and then some.

You don't need to put on weight as you age. That is the basic yet progressive commitment of The Entire Body Reset, which uncovers why standard eating routine and exercise guidance quits working for us as we approach midlife — and uncovers how straightforward changes to the manner in which we eat can stop, and, surprisingly, switch, age-related weight gain and muscle misfortune.

The Entire Body Reset presents shocking new proof about the force of "protein timing" for individuals at midlife — research that blows away flow government rules, disproves the fantasy of easing back digestion systems and "unavoidable" weight gain, and meaningfully impacts the way individuals in their mid-forties and more established ought to ponder food. The Entire Body Reset makes sense of in straightforward, moving terms precisely the way that our bodies change with age, and how eating to oblige those changes can cause us to answer practice as though we were twenty to thirty years more youthful.

Introduction

An extensive body resharp, short for "extensive body reshaping," refers to a comprehensive process of transforming the physical appearance of one's body through various means. This procedure typically involves a combination of diet, exercise, and potentially medical interventions, depending on the individual's goals and circumstances.

The process of an extensive body resharp often begins with setting specific goals for the desired physical transformation. These goals can include elements like weight loss, muscle gain, improvement in overall fitness, or achieving a more proportionate body shape . It is essential to establish realistic and attainable objectives to create a sustainable and healthy transformation.

Diet plays a crucial role in an extensive body resharp. It usually involves modifying one's eating habits to support weight loss or muscle gain, depending on the desired outcome. This may incorporate calorie restriction, macronutrient adjustments, and an emphasis on consuming nutrient-dense foods. Consulting with a registered dietitian can be helpful in developing a tailored diet plan suited to an individual's specific needs and goals.

Exercise is another fundamental aspect of an extensive body resharp. It involves engaging in regular physical activity to stimulate muscle growth, improve cardiovascular health, enhance overall fitness, and aid in weight loss. This can involve a combination of cardiovascular exercises, strength training, flexibility training, and other targeted workouts to address specific body areas.

Depending on the individual's circumstances and desired results, medical interventions may also be considered as part of an extensive body resharp. This can include procedures such as liposuction to remove stubborn fat deposits, breast augmentation or reduction, abdominoplast(commonly known as a tummy tuck), or other body contouring surgeries. It is crucial to consult with a qualified medical professional to discuss the potential risks, benefits, and suitability of such interventions.

Throughout the process of an extensive body resharp, it is essential to prioritize overall health and well-being. It is advisable to work with a team of professionals, including nutritionists, personal trainers, and medical experts, to ensure a safe and effective transformation. Moreover, maintaining a positive mindset, practicing self-care, and establishing realistic expectations are key to achieving long-term success and sustained results.

1:"The Age-Defying Magic of Protein Timing"

tells the story of two different approaches to a healthy diet, focusing on the role of protein in maintaining youthfulness and vitality. It emphasizes the importance of not just what we eat but also when we eat.

The first diet follows the traditional approach where protein is consumed evenly throughout the day. This diet involves regular meals with protein-rich foods like chicken, fish, dairy, and legumes. While this approach provides the necessary nutrients, it fails to take advantage of the body's natural cycles and its ability to optimize protein absorption.

The second diet, on the other hand, incorporates a concept known as protein timing. This approach recognizes that our bodies have specific windows of time when they are more receptive to protein intake for muscle repair, growth, and overall health. By strategically timing protein intake, this diet maximizes the benefits and slows down the aging process.

The story highlights how the second diet, with its emphasis on protein timing, produces better results in terms of maintaining muscle mass, reducing body fat, and increasing energy levels. It also explores the scientific research and studies that support this concept, specifically focusing on the role of protein synthesis and its impact on aging.

Through this narrative, "The Age-Defying Magic of Protein Timing" encourages readers to rethink their approach to nutrition and consider incorporating protein timing into their daily lives. It emphasizes the importance of understanding our bodies' natural rhythms and capitalizing on them for optimal health and longevity.

Protein consumption and its association with changes in body composition, muscle function and different strategies to optimize the muscle protein synthetic response have received considerable attention. However, we are not aware of any epidemiological study examining the time-of-day consumption (afternoon versus evening) of protein on strength and lean mass. The purpose was to examine the associations between afternoon and evening protein consumption, at different protein thresholds (i.e. 15, 20, 25 and 30 g), in relation to leg lean mass and knee extensor strength in men. Dietary protein consumption was assessed using 24-h dietary interview format. Knee extensor strength was measured on an isokinetic dynamometer. Leg lean mass was estimated from whole-body DXA scans. Participants who consumed 20 g, 25 g and 30 g of protein in the evening had greater leg lean mass than those who consumed protein in the afternoon ($P<0.05$). However, there was no difference in leg lean mass for 15 g of protein consumption in the evening compared to the afternoon ($P>0.05$). For strength, there were no differences between evening and afternoon consumption of protein for 15 g, 20 g or 25 g ($P>0.05$); however, those consuming at least 30 g of protein in the evening had greater knee extensor strength compared to those consuming similar amounts in the afternoon ($P = 0.05$). These findings suggest that evening protein consumption is associated with greater leg lean mass and knee extensor strength when compared to afternoon protein consumption. Based on these findings, we cautiously hypothesize that there may be a circadian rhythm in muscle protein metabolism.

In January everyone wants to be fit and lose weight so I decided to dive into what you need to know about protein amounts for weight loss and protein timing.

"How much protein should I eat, and how should I divide that throughout the day?" This is one big question I always get. Out of the three macronutrients – carbohydrates, protein and fat – protein is the key for weight loss, and protein timing makes a big difference. Now there are three reasons for that:

1. Protein takes longer to digest than the other macronutrients.
2. As you lose weight you will most likely lose muscle.
3. Protein helps control your hunger hormone ghrelin.

Protein Digestion and How it Impacts Weight Loss

The body takes a while to digest the matrix of the protein, so the protein sits in your stomach for a longer time. This is one way that it helps to control your hunger. By spreading out meals and snacks throughout the day, you're helping to control satiety and cravings from not eating for too long.

Weight Loss and Losing Muscle

As you lose weight you most likely will lose muscle as well and therefore, we must prevent that from happening because muscle drives your metabolism

If you lose weight and you're losing muscle, by the end you're going to have a low metabolism. That's another reason you want to add protein to your meals.

Hunger Hormone Ghrelin

What is Ghrelin?

Ghrelin is a hormone in your gut refered to as the "hunger hormone" because it's role is to increase your hunger.

Ghrelin Hormone Function.

Ghrelin fights you and wants you to stay at homeostasis. It doesn't want you to lose the weight and the hormone actually increases as you lose weight. Everyone who is losing weight is hungrier because they're cutting calories and likely not eating enough protein. So, by adding protein, you can help control the hunger hormone ghrelin and keep your hunger hormone in check.

How Much Protein to Eat Per Meal

The main target of protein per meal is 30-40g (lower end for females, higher end for males). If you eat more than that, your body cannot utilize it. You won't metabolize it the same so, it's wasted. To maximize your weight loss, metabolism, and protein, target 30-40g.

For snacks, I typically recommend aiming for 10-20g.

Protein Timing

The goal is to eat every 3-4 hours. Ghrelin comes back by the fourth hour, so if you don't eat frequently, ghrelin can make someone eat 40% more without even knowing it.

Sample Protein Timing for 1500 Calories Per Day

Here are sample meals and how to divide protein throughout the day for proper protein timing.

Meal	Food	Amount of

		Protein
Breakfast (6am)	Egg Muffins with Spinach (2 for female; 3 for male) 1 cup of blueberries 1 glass of milk	30-40g from the eggs and milk
Snack (9am)	Greek yogurt parfait with mango and pecans	~10-20g from the Greek yogurt and pecans
Lunch (12pm)	Panini with turkey, cheese Small green smoothie	30-40g from all items
Snack (4pm)	**Option 1:** Two	~10-20g from

	hardboiled eggs, apple **Option 2:** Smoothie with Greek yogurt, milk, protein powder and frozen strawberries	eggs ~20 from yogurt, milk, protein powder
	Option 1: High protein pasta with meat sauce and cheese on top. **Option 2 (vegan/vegetarian):**Soup with lima beans and rice protein	30-40g protein

	powder	
Dessert	15-30g of 70% dark chocolate (~1-2 squares) and several pieces of dried fruit (apricots, figs, prunes)	

2:Our Changing Bodies, Our Changing Needs

The food we eat gives our bodies the information and fuel it needs to properly function. If it does not get the right information, our metabolic processes can suffer and our health can decline. It is essential to have good nutrition based on healthy eating habits to enable you to stay healthy, active, and live a longer life.

In short, the nutrition you put in your body can help you avoid certain diseases that can put your life at risk and cause your health to deteriorate.

How does food affect our bodies?

The nutrients from the food we put in our bodies give our cells the ability to perform their necessary functions. Think of it as planting a garden. If you are planting a tomato seed, ideally you use the right soil and the right amount of sun for the best success. However, if you use the cheapest dirt and don't give it enough sunlight you may still get a tomato, but the tomato may not be the ripest, roundest, reddest, or tastiest tomato.

In other words, giving our bodies the right nutrients can help you grow to a healthier version of yourself. Thinking about food from this aspect goes beyond calories and good food versus bad food. You need to focus on the foods you are putting in your body versus the foods you are excluding. Look at food as a way to fuel your body and help fight.

Nutrition and disease

When we eat food it goes through a digestive process. Part of this process involves absorbing vitamins and minerals from that food and distributing it into the bloodstream which leads to the blood vessels, coronary arteries, and the heart muscle.

Depending on what types of food you are eating can cause your heart to pump harder and exert more energy. This could eventually lead to heart failure and a heart attack.

Your sodium intake plays a major role in affecting your heart rate and blood pressure. By consuming salty foods, your body will retain water to dilute the blood volume. This causes more blood to circulate throughout your body and your heart to work harder.

The recommended sodium intake by the Centers for Disease Control and Prevention is 180 – 500 mg of sodium a day. However, Americans on average consume over 3,400 mg of sodium a day. Most of these are pre-prepared and processed foods.

A diet that is high in saturated and trans fats will elevate your bad cholesterol (LDL) and could lead to the hardening of arteries and plaque forming on the inner linings of blood vessels which will further narrow them. The narrowed openings mean that as the heart receives the blood it must work harder to maintain blood flow in order to pump blood through the narrowed channels.

Similarly, if you are not maintaining a healthy diet this could increase your risk for various cancers. According to a study published in 2018 by The BMJ, a study was performed on the amount of processing and the amount of change the ingredients go through to help improve flavor, coloring, and shelf life. It was found that for every 10% increase in consumption of ultra-processed foods was associated with a 12% higher risk for cancer in general and an 11% increased risk for breast cancer.

While these foods can cause harm there are foods that can help improve your health and heart function. Healthy fats such as olive oil and whole grains can help lower your cholesterol and help prevent plaque from forming in the arteries. By improving the blood flow, your heart will be able to pump blood easier causing less strain and stress on your heart which could eventually lower your heart rate.

What is poor nutrition

By depriving our bodies of the nourishment it needs can lead to poor nutrition and eating habits which can cause obesity, diabetes, and increase certain risk factors for stroke, heart disease, and cancer.

Poor nutrition is caused by putting the wrong types of food in your body that do not have the nutrients that we need most. These foods include ones that are low in fiber and vitamins or are high in fat, sugar, and salt. While many of the packaged foods we purchase at the grocery store meet our taste bud requirements, the way these are packaged and stored may strip the food of the nutrients our body requires and eliminate your chance of healthy weight loss.

Poor nutrition can also be caused by overeating. If you are taking in more calories than you are burning each day, even if these are the "right" foods, can eventually cause weight gain and lead to obesity. If you suffer from being overweight or obese, this can lead to diabetes and heart problems.

On the other hand, if you are undereating you could be depriving your body of the nutrients it needs. Those who suffer from diseases such as anorexia or bulimia are just as much in jeopardy of heart complications and disease as those who overeat.

If you are concerned about the number of calories you are putting in your body it is best to discuss with your doctor or nutrition and dietetics expert.

How does poor nutrition affect you?

Poor nutrition can affect your health in many ways, not only can it lead to certain diseases but it can also affect your mental health, energy levels, complexion, and your overall well being. In the short term, poor nutrition can contribute to stress, tiredness, and our capacity to work. Furthermore, it can lead to:

- being overweight or obese
- tooth decay
- high blood pressure
- high cholesterol
- heart disease and stroke
- type-2 diabetes
- osteoporosis
- some cancers

- depression
- eating disorders,

- Poor nutrition can impair your daily health and

- wellbeing and reduce your

- ability to lead an enjoyable active life.

- **Healthy eating habit**

We've all been told that healthy eating can transform your life and help you live a longer and more active one. But what does healthy eating actually mean and how do you start putting this into practice and breaking bad habits? For some, this may be a way to help them lose weight, for others the goal may be to lower their blood pressure, and for others, it may just be to have a healthier way of living.

This transformation doesn't happen overnight. You can't just wake up on Sunday morning and break all of your bad habits without the cravings. This is a gradual process and can be as simple as choosing steamed broccoli as a side instead of loaded mashed potatoes. Or choosing an apple over chips for your mid-morning snack.

Here are some helpful tips and ideas that will soon have you well on the way to bursting with health and vitality:

    a. Get more fruits and veggies in your day. Start your morning with a bowl of oatmeal and some blueberries. Aim for two servings of fruit and five servings of veggies each day.

    b. Eat less saturated and trans fats. Read the labels for the products you are purchasing. You may be surprised at the ingredients and opt for a different brand.

c. Eat less salt. Make a conscious effort to put less and less salt on your food, until just a dash is all you need.

d.Eat less sugar. Try substituting honey in your coffee and opt for less sugary desserts. For instance, if you are craving dessert, try blending frozen bananas and topping it some strawberries.

Drink more water and aim for drinking half your body weight in ounces. Choosing water over sugary drinks can help you lose weight, clear your complexion, and, since our bodies are made up of 70% water, you may feel healthier all around.

Check your portions. Fill half of your dinner plate with a variety of vegetables or salad, add lean protein foods such as meat, fish, chicken or legumes (chickpeas, lentils, kidney beans etc) to take up a quarter of the plate, last add in grain foods such as rice, pasta or noodles to take up the remaining quarter of the plate.

Plan ahead. One of the main reasons people end up eating fast food or a bag of chips is because they are in a rush. Plan out your meals on the weekends, including your snacks, and purchase only what you need and prep your food.

3. Let's Spend a Day on The Whole Body Reset!(A 7-Day Whole Body Reset Sample Menu)

Day 1:

•Breakfast: Fresh fruit salad with Greek yogurt

•Snack: Mixed nuts

•Lunch: Grilled chicken breast with steamed vegetables

•Snack: Carrot sticks with hummus

•Dinner: Baked salmon with quinoa and roasted asparagus

•Dessert: Chia seed pudding with berries

Day 2:

•Breakfast: Veggie omelette with whole wheat toast

•Snack: Apple slices with almond butter

•Lunch: Lentil soup with a side salad

•Snack: Rice cakes with avocado spread

•Dinner: Quinoa-stuffed bell peppers

•Dessert: Dark chocolate squares

Day 3:

•Breakfast: Overnight oats with berries and almond milk

•Snack: Celery sticks with peanut butter

•Lunch: Grilled shrimp salad with mixed greens•

Snacks: Greek yogurt with honey

•Dinner: Baked chicken thigh with roasted sweet potatoes and green beans

•Dessert: Fresh fruit kebabs

Day 4:

•Breakfast: Spinach and mushroom scrambled eggs

•Snack: Homemade trail mix

•Lunch: Quinoa salad with cherry tomatoes and cucumber

•Snack: Edamame beans

•Dinner: Oven-roasted cod with quinoa and steamed broccoli

•Dessert: Banana "nice cream"

Day 5:

•Breakfast: Protein smoothie with spinach, banana, and almond milk

•Snack: Sliced bell peppers with hummus

•Lunch: Grilled tofu with roasted vegetables

•Snack: Cottage cheese with cucumber slices

•Dinner: Grilled steak with roasted sweet potato fries and mixed greens

•Dessert: Frozen grapes

Day 6:•Breakfast: Avocado toast with poached eggs

•Snack: Kale chips

•Lunch: Chickpea salad with tomatoes and feta cheese

•Snack: Protein shake

•Dinner: Baked salmon with quinoa pilaf and steamed asparagus

•Dessert: Greek yogurt with granola

Day 7:•Breakfast: Quinoa breakfast bowl with mixed berries and nuts

•Snack: Apple slices with cottage cheese

•Lunch: Turkey wrap with lettuce, tomato, and avocado

•Snack: Rice cakes with almond butter

•Dinner: Grilled chicken with roasted vegetables and brown rice

•Dessert: Mixed berry smoothie

Remember, this is just a sample menu, and you can customize it according to your preferences and dietary restrictions. It's always a good idea to consult with a nutritionist or healthcare professional before making any decisions.

4:The Six Simple Secrets of Better   health muscle-Building Foods for Vegans.

Striking the right balance between <u>protein</u>, <u>carbs</u> and fats with the right amount calories is <u>muscle food</u> 101, but making sure you are setting your body up for success with the correct micronutrients to foster a <u>muscle building</u> furnace, can make it a lot easier.

While the ultimate fate of those calories is decided largely by how much you burn day to day, genetics and various lifestyle factors have a say, too. The amount and intensity of your <u>workout</u> will also be impacted by the quality of your <u>diet</u>. It's difficult to push yourself when you're feeling lethargic.

For example, missing out on vitamin E can cause muscle weakness and leg cramps, while inadequate vitamin A intake can result in dizziness, nausea, muscle and joint pain, and even loss of balance. Not conducive to a PB-crushing leg sesh.

You might already be regularly munching some of the foods below, others may come as a surprise – but trust us, all of them will fuel your mission to build lean muscle. Load up your shopping trolley with our best muscle building food picks.

1. Whole eggs

Another day, another article touting the benefits of eggs. Those golden orbs contain large amounts of the amino acid leucine, which is essential for post-exercise muscle recovery. Whole eggs in particular are considered to be something of a protein synthesis powerhouse. In fact, eating whole eggs after a workout elicits a 40 per cent greater muscle-building response than consuming egg whites alone, a study published in *The American Journal of Clinical Nutrition* found.

2. Salmon

As well as a huge helping of complete protein(around 20g per 100g serve), salmon is high in omega-3 fatty acids EPA and DHA, which optimise nutrient partitioning by reducing inflammation. Omega-3 increases insulin sensitivity, a study from Harvard University found, resulting in less insulin floating around in your bloodstream. A good thing, because insulin boosts fat storage. Just try to avoid reheating it in the office microwave.

3. Soy beans

Gracing third place in our list of best muscle building foods, soy beans could boost your plant based muscle gains. If your goal is building lean, green muscle, soybeans are your most dependable option. Unlike other vegetarian sources of protein, those little legumes contain all nine essential amino acids, making them an essential vegan muscle food. Tofu, tempeh, and most vegetarian meat alternatives are made out of soy, which boasts 36 grams per 100g serve.around.

4. Pineapple

Fruit isn't your a-typical bodybuilding fare, but an exception can be made for pineapple. It's the only food known to contain bromelein, an enzyme that digests protein. Fun fact: pineapple is often uncomfortable to eat because the bromelain is digesting the skin on the inside of your mouth. Plus, its anti-inflammatory properties will help soothe post-workout pain, tenderness and swelling.

5. Greek yogurt

As well as being loaded with fast-digesting whey protein and slow-digesting casein protein – around 10 grams total per 100g serve – Greek yogurt is a source of vitamin D, which helps your body absorb calcium and phosphorus. Calcium is crucial for muscle contractions, while phosphorus is essential for creating ATP (the form of energy your body uses). According to research by Baylor University, a mix of whey and casein protein is the optimum combination for increasing lean mass.

6. Garlic

Your co-workers may not thank you, but your biceps will. In a study published in *The Journal of Nutrition*, garlic was shown to increase testosterone and lower cortisol in rats on a high-protein diet. How? It's all to do with a compound within garlic called allicin, which reduces the amount of 'stress hormone' pumping around your body. Cortisol competes with testosterone in your muscle cells, so essentially less stress results in better gains.

7. Turkey breast

We're all well aware of the high protein content that turkey possesses, at 29 grams of protein per 100g, turkey is another big protein hitter. But this lean meat has another superpower in relation to the special mineral it contains. Turkey contains 30mg of magnesium per 100 grams making it an impressive addition to your health promoting meal plan. Low levels of magnesium can cause muscle cramps and have been linked to depression according to a <u>review</u> published by *Pharmacological Reports*. It's also high in zinc, which supports protein synthesis and helps your body maintain healthy levels of testosterone, as mentioned by researchers at the <u>Wayne State University School of Medicine</u> in Michigan, US.

8. Kidney beans

Being higher in carbohydrates, beans and legumes are often overlooked for their leaner cousins. But these fibrous foods are essential for a healthy gut – something you depend on to absorb the nutrients, minerals and supplements required to carve lean muscle. Kidney beans contain the most, with around

8 grams of protein per 100g serve (and around 10 grams of fibre!). Pair them with a whole grain such as brown rice to make a complete protein.

9. Tuna

Inexpensive and versatile, tuna packs around 25 grams of protein per 100g serve, making it hearty muscle-building fare – with the added benefit of those essential omega-3 fatty acids. Just don't make it the only thing you eat, or you could wind up with some unwanted side effects. Like mercury poisoning.

10. Lean beef

Muscle food of the bovine variety has come under fire in recent years, but enjoyed in moderation, it can make meaningful gym fuel. As well as 26 grams of protein per 100g, which is around the size of a hamburger patty, lean beef contains high levels of zinc. This nutrient is important for testosterone production and also helps your body to recover quicker from exercise.

11. Extra virgin olive oil

The monounsaturated fats in olive oil stimulate protein production for muscle growth and prevent tissue breakdown, but the Mediterranean favourite also has some hidden muscle benefits. It increases insulin sensitivity in your muscles, allowing them to make optimal use of glucose, amino acids and nutrients. Olive oil also contains oleuropein – a phenolic compound that causes white fat cells to act like brown fat cells, according to researchers at Kobe Women's University in Japan.

12. Cottage cheese

Cottage cheese contains the slow-digesting protein casein, which explains why people like to eat it before bed. Sleep repairs your muscles up to a point; after a few hours a fasting element kicks in, and your body begins breaking muscles down to use as energy. Cottage cheese allows for a sustained release of amino acids throughout the night. Plus with 15 grams of protein and just 85 calories per 100g serve, it's a muscle food no-brainer.

13.Prawns

Prawns pack a protein punch of 20 grams per 100 grams, making it the perfect choice of muscle building foods. According to an articlepublished by the *Shellfish Association of Great Britain,* you can get 47% of your RDA of B12 from just 100 grams which will help prevent anemia, osteoporosis and support your memory.

14.Oats

Oats are a perfect post workout food to replenish your muscles with the energy they need to ensure you adequately recover and are ready to power through your next workout. Aside from the energy they give you, oats are a unique grain with as much as 11 grams of protein per 100 grams. Plus, if you struggle with digestive issues, something that can be most unwelcome during training sessions, oats are packed with 10 grams of fibre per 100 grams to help you avoid any unpleasant issues.

15.Peas

Peas are an underrated source of muscle building protein and muscle fuelling starch. With 14 grams of carbs and 5 grams of protein per 100 grams, the impressive protein and carb combo sets the perfect muscle gain environment post workout. According to an article published by the *Cambridge University Press,* the vitamin and mineral contents of peas may play important roles in the prevention of illnesses. Pair them with rice and beans and you have a full spectrum of amino acids (the building blocks for building muscle).

5: The Inside Story of Your Gut

The gut, also known as the gastrointestinal tract, is a complex system that plays a crucial role in our overall health and well-being. It is often referred to as the "second brain" because it contains a vast network of nerves that communicate with the brain and influence our mood, emotions, and even our behavior.

Inside the gut, there are trillions of microorganisms, including bacteria, viruses, fungi, and other microbes, collectively known as the gut microbiota. These tiny organisms live in a symbiotic relationship with our bodies, helping us digest food, produce essential nutrients, and support a healthy immune system.

The gut microbiota is incredibly diverse and unique to each individual, much like a fingerprint. It is influenced by various factors, including genetics, diet, lifestyle, and environmental exposures. A balanced and diverse gut microbiota is associated with good health, while an imbalance, known as dysbiosis, can lead to various digestive disorders, metabolic conditions, and even mental health disorders.

The gut also produces and houses a wide array of hormones, neurotransmitters, and other molecules that regulate appetite, metabolism, and other physiological processes. For example, around 90% of the neurotransmitter serotonin, which is involved in regulating mood, is produced in the gut.

Maintaining a healthy gut is crucial for overall well-being. Eating a balanced diet rich in fiber, prebiotics (food for beneficial gut bacteria), and fermented foods can promote a diverse gut microbiota. Regular exercise, stress management, and adequate sleep also play important roles in gut health.
Understanding the intricate workings of our gut can empower us to make informed
choices about our diet and lifestyle that can positively impact our physical and mental health.

6: How The Whole Body Reset Can Help Fight Disease and Save Your Life (Over and Over Again)

The Whole Body Reset is a comprehensive approach to improving health and fighting disease. It aims to reset the body at a cellular level, optimizing its natural functions and defenses. By adopting healthy lifestyle habits and making conscious choices about nutrition, exercise, sleep, stress management, and mindfulness, individuals can support their body's ability to fight disease and improve overall well-being. The Whole Body Reset is a repetitive process that individuals can follow throughout their lives to maintain optimal health and potentially increase longevity.

The whole body reset can be beneficial in fighting disease and promoting longevity in several ways:

1.Enhancing immune function: A healthy immune system is crucial in defending the body against various infections and diseases. By following a whole body reset, you can strengthen your immune system by providing it with the necessary nutrients, reducing inflammation, and improving overall health.

2.Reducing inflammation: Chronic inflammation is associated with the development of various diseases, including cardiovascular diseases, diabetes, and certain types of cancer. A whole body reset emphasizes an anti-inflammatory diet, which can reduce inflammation and support overall health.

3.Supporting gut health: The gut plays a vital role in our overall health, including digestion, nutrient absorption, and even immune function. A whole body reset promotes a healthy gut by incorporating prebiotic and probiotic-rich foods, reducing processed foods, and managing stress levels, which can impact gut health.

4.Balancing hormones: Hormonal imbalances can contribute to various health issues, such as weight gain, mood swings, and reproductive problems. By adopting a whole body reset, you can support hormone balance through proper nutrition, exercise, stress management, and adequate sleep.

5.Managing weight: Excess weight is a risk factor for many chronic diseases, including heart disease, diabetes, and certain cancers. A whole body reset focuses on adopting a balanced and nutrient-dense diet, regular exercise, and healthy lifestyle choices, which can help manage weight and improve overall health.

6.Promoting overall well-being: A whole body reset is not just about physical health; it also encompasses mental and emotional well-being. By making lifestyle changes such as practicing mindfulness, engaging in regular exercise, and getting adequate sleep, you can improve your overall well-being and reduce the risk of various diseases.

By implementing a whole body reset, you can address multiple aspects of your health simultaneously, which can have a positive impact on your overall quality of life and longevity. However, it's important to note that everyone's needs may differ, and it is always a good idea to consult with a healthcare professional before making significant changes to your lifestyle.

7:Your Whole Body Fitness Plan

The Whole Body Fitness Plan is a comprehensive approach to improving and maintaining overall physical fitness. It focuses on addressing various aspects of fitness, including cardiovascular endurance, muscular strength and endurance, flexibility, and body composition. Here's a breakdown of the key components of the plan:

1. **Cardiovascular Endurance**: This aspect of fitness targets the health of your heart and lungs. It involves activities that increase your heart rate and breathing rate sustained over a period. Examples include jogging, swimming, cycling, or participating in aerobic classes.

2. **Muscular Strength and Endurance**: This component aims to strengthen and tone your muscles while also improving their ability to perform repetitive tasks. It typically involves resistance training exercises like weightlifting, bodyweight exercises, or using resistance bands.

3. **Flexibility: Flexibility** exercises help improve joint range of motion and prevent stiffness or injury. They include stretching exercises, yoga, or Pilates.

Maintaining good flexibility can enhance overall performance and reduce the risk of muscle imbalances.

4. Body Composition: This refers to the ratio of lean body mass (muscle, bone, organs) to body fat. To improve body composition, the plan may incorporate strategies like a balanced diet, calorie control, and a combination of aerobic exercise and strength training.

5:Rest and Recovery: Adequate rest and recovery are crucial for your body to repair and grow stronger. Make sure to include rest days in your fitness plan to allow your muscles to recover and prevent overtraining.

6:Core Exercises: Working on your core muscles is important for stability and balance. Core exercises, such as planks, crunches, or twists, strengthen the muscles in your abdomen, lower back, and hips.

In addition to these components, the Whole Body Fitness Plan may include other factors such as proper nutrition, hydration, rest, and recovery. It's important to tailor the plan to individual needs and goals, considering factors like age, fitness level, and any underlying health conditions.

Working with a professional fitness trainer or consulting a healthcare professional can help design a personalized plan that suits your specific requirements and ensures a safe and effective fitness journey.

Remember, it's always a good idea to consult with a fitness professional or trainer to help you develop a customized whole body fitness plan that suits your specific needs and goals.

8: The Metabolism Myth

The Metabolism Myth is a common misconception that many people believe regarding weight loss and body composition. It suggests that people with a slow metabolism are doomed to struggle with weight gain and find it much harder to lose weight compared to those with a faster metabolism. However, it is essential to understand that metabolism is a complex process that varies from person to person, and its impact on weight loss is often overstated.

Metabolism refers to the chemical reactions that occur in the body to convert food into energy. It is influenced by several factors, such as age, genetics, body composition, hormone levels, and lifestyle choices. While it's true that some individuals may have naturally faster or slower metabolisms, the difference in overall calorie expenditure between these individuals is usually quite small.

Weight gain or loss is primarily determined by the balance between calorie intake and expenditure. If you consume more calories than your body needs, regardless of your metabolism rate, you are likely to gain weight. On the other hand, if you consume fewer calories than your body requires, you are likely to lose weight.

The key to successful weight management lies in adopting a balanced and sustainable approach that includes a healthy diet, regular physical activity, adequate sleep, and managing stress levels. Focusing solely on metabolism as the determining factor can often lead to unrealistic expectations and disappointment when trying to achieve weight loss goals.

While there are certain medical conditions that can influence metabolism, the majority of individuals can maintain a healthy weight through an active and mindful lifestyle. Rather than getting fixated on the metabolism myth, it is more productive to concentrate on maintaining a balanced diet, engaging in regular exercise, and listening to your body's hunger and fullness cues.

Remember, sustainable weight loss is a gradual process that requires patience, consistency, and habits that can be maintained in the long term. Consulting with a healthcare professional or a registered dietitian can also provide valuable guidance and personalized advice on managing weight effectively.

In conclusion

The extensive body reshaping process is an innovative approach to enhancing one's physical appearance. By combining advanced surgical techniques with a comprehensive
understanding of individual goals and desires, this procedure offers individuals the opportunity to transform their bodies and boost their self-confidence. Whether it involves sculpting the abdomen, thighs, arms, or other areas, extensive body reshaping can produce remarkable results. However, it is essential to approach this process with realistic expectations, proper consultation with a qualified professional, and a commitment to maintaining a healthy lifestyle post-surgery. Ultimately, extensive body reshaping has the potential to empower individuals and provide them with a renewed sense of self that aligns with their body image.